Easy steps to fight against obesity

Strategies for sustainable weight loss and unlocking the secret of balanced nutrition

Javier F. Williams

Table of contents

Chapter 1: Introduction

Obesity stands as a prevailing challenge in our modern society, impacting individuals and communities alike. In this introduction, we embark on a journey to unravel the complexities of obesity, exploring its implications on health and well-being. As we delve into this topic, our aim is not only to comprehend the gravity of the issue but also to provide a glimpse into a transformative path – a series of easy steps designed to bring about positive change.

Understanding Obesity Today

At the core of our exploration lies the need to comprehend the multifaceted nature of obesity. It's more than just a number on a scale; it's a condition intricately woven into the fabric of our lifestyles, genetics, and environment. We dissect the medical aspects, examining how excess weight can lead to various health issues such as cardiovascular diseases, diabetes, and a myriad of other complications. Understanding the science behind obesity becomes the foundation upon which our journey toward effective solutions is built.

Yet, our exploration goes beyond the clinical definitions. We delve into the societal aspects, acknowledging the challenges individuals face in a world where unhealthy food options are abundant, sedentary lifestyles are prevalent, and societal norms sometimes perpetuate unhealthy habits. By understanding the broader context, we empower ourselves to confront not only the physical manifestations of obesity but also the underlying contributors that shape our choices.

A Sneak Peek into Easy Steps for Change

As we navigate the landscape of combating obesity, we offer readers a preview of what lies ahead – a roadmap of easy steps carefully crafted to initiate positive transformation. These steps are not about drastic, unsustainable changes; instead, they represent a collection of manageable adjustments designed to fit seamlessly into everyday life.

Our approach is rooted in the belief that sustainable change is born from simplicity. Each step is a building block, a small change that, when combined with others, forms a powerful foundation for a healthier lifestyle. The sneak peek serves as an invitation, enticing readers to join us on this journey toward better health, assuring them that the path to change can be not only effective but also accessible.

In the upcoming chapters, we will explore the core principles of nutrition simplified for success, delve into the importance of movement without overwhelming workouts, master the art of mindful eating, recognize the significance of hydration, and navigate social situations with smart choices. Additionally, we will uncover the power of a support system, recognizing that the journey toward a healthier lifestyle is often more fulfilling when shared.

In essence, this introduction serves as a gateway into a realm of possibilities. It invites readers to reconsider their relationship with health, presenting a narrative where positive change is not only achievable but also enjoyable. As we embark on this exploration together, we encourage each reader to embrace the potential for transformation, recognizing that the journey to fight against obesity can indeed be paved with easy and sustainable steps.

Chapter 2: Demystifying Obesity

In our contemporary world, where lifestyles evolve at a rapid pace, obesity stands as a complex and often misunderstood challenge. This essay aims to demystify the intricate layers of obesity, define its profound impact on health and society, and underscore the urgent need for personal action.

Demystifying Obesity:

Obesity goes beyond a mere body weight issue; it's a multifaceted condition influenced by genetics, environment, and lifestyle. Contrary to simplistic judgments, it requires a nuanced understanding. The Body Mass Index (BMI) classification, while a useful metric, merely scratches the surface of this intricate health concern. By unraveling the various factors contributing to obesity, we can dispel myths and foster a more compassionate perspective.

Defining Obesity and Its Impact:

Delving into the health realm, obesity emerges as a catalyst for a myriad of serious conditions. From the insidious infiltration of cardiovascular diseases to the looming threat of diabetes, its impact reverberates through individual lives and extends its reach to the societal level. The economic burden on healthcare systems becomes apparent, creating a web of challenges that necessitate comprehensive solutions. Global statistics and poignant studies serve as a stark reminder of the urgency to address this pervasive issue.

The Urgency for Personal Action:

Amidst the statistics and medical jargon, the core of the issue lies in personal responsibility. The urgency to address and prevent obesity calls for a reevaluation of individual lifestyles. Balanced nutrition and regular physical activity emerge as crucial pillars in this journey towards wellness. Education and awareness become powerful tools, empowering individuals to make informed choices and break free from the cycle of unhealthy habits.

this exploration into obesity's layers, impact, and the call for personal action is not just an academic exercise; it's a call to introspection and change. By demystifying the complexities, defining the gravity of its consequences, and emphasizing personal agency, we pave the way for a healthier future—one where the layers of obesity are gradually peeled away to reveal the path to wellness.

Chapter 3: The Core Principles

The Core Principles (Obesity)," we delve into the critical aspects of addressing and preventing obesity through simplified nutrition strategies. This chapter is designed to provide practical insights into navigating nutrition for success, with a particular focus on combating obesity through effective portion control.

Obesity, a prevalent health concern, is often linked to lifestyle choices, including diet. This chapter aims to shed light on core principles that simplify nutrition and contribute to obesity prevention and management.

1. Holistic Approach to Nutrition

A holistic approach to nutrition involves understanding that combating obesity extends beyond calorie counting. It encompasses making informed choices about the types of foods consumed, their nutritional value, and the impact on overall health. By embracing a holistic mindset, individuals can tailor their diets to support weight management.

2. *Identifying Culprits: Sugars and Processed Foods*

Recognizing the role of sugars and processed foods in obesity is crucial. The chapter explores the harmful effects of excessive sugar consumption and the hidden additives in processed foods. Empowering readers with knowledge about these culprits enables them to make healthier food choices and combat obesity at its roots.

Simplifying Nutrition for Success

1. Balanced Diet for Obesity Prevention

The foundation of the chapter lies in promoting a balanced diet as a key element in preventing and managing obesity. Emphasizing the importance of including a variety of nutrient-dense foods, such as fruits, vegetables, lean proteins, and whole grains, encourages readers to adopt a sustainable and health-focused approach to nutrition.

2. Nutritional Education

Providing nutritional education is a vital component of simplifying nutrition for success. Understanding the nutritional content of different foods empowers individuals to make informed choices. The chapter delves into essential nutrients, their sources, and their roles in supporting overall health, creating a knowledge base for effective dietary decisions.

Practical Tips for Portion Control

1. Portion Control and Obesity

Portion control is a key strategy in combating obesity. This section of the chapter focuses on practical tips to help individuals manage their portions effectively. By adopting these strategies, readers can develop a healthier relationship with food, leading to sustained weight management.

2. **Mindful Eating Practices**

Encouraging mindful eating practices is integral to effective portion control. The chapter explores techniques such as eating slowly, savoring each bite, and paying attention to hunger and fullness cues. By incorporating mindfulness into their eating habits, individuals can avoid overeating and make more conscious food choices.

3. **Meal Planning for Weight Management**

The chapter highlights the significance of meal planning in the context of obesity prevention. Offering practical tips for structuring well-balanced meals, it guides readers in creating a sustainable meal plan that supports weight management goals. This includes preparing meals with appropriate portion sizes and nutritional content.

4. **Behavioral Strategies**

Understanding the behavioral aspects of eating is crucial for those combating obesity. The chapter introduces strategies such as recognizing emotional triggers for overeating, finding alternative coping mechanisms, and building healthier habits. By addressing the psychological components of eating, individuals can make lasting changes in their relationship with food.

The Core Principles (Obesity) by simplifying nutrition for success and providing practical tips for portion control. By embracing a holistic approach to nutrition, understanding the role of sugars and processed foods, and focusing on balanced meals, individuals can navigate their journey towards preventing and managing obesity. Practical tips for portion control, coupled with mindful eating practices and behavioral strategies, empower readers to make informed choices, fostering a healthier lifestyle and sustained weight management.

Chapter 4: Move, Groove, and Improve

In the journey toward a healthier lifestyle, the importance of embracing everyday physical activity cannot be overstated. This chapter serves as a comprehensive guide, outlining strategies to combat obesity by making movement an integral part of daily life. We delve into the transformative power of finding your exercise bliss, encouraging a shift from viewing exercise as a chore to embracing it as a source of joy and well-being.

Hope you're enjoying reading this book?

Are you a victim of syphilis or your family and friends **"Syphilis and Its Nutritional Guide."** This compelling book goes beyond conventional wisdom, offering a unique perspective on managing syphilis through the lens of nutrition. Packed with practical tips, it's your roadmap to wellness. Don't just survive; thrive with the power of informed choices. Grab your copy now and take control of your health narrative.

CLICK HERE TO GET SYPHILIS AND ITS NUTRITIONAL GUIDE

The Epidemic of Obesity

Obesity has become a global health concern, affecting millions of lives and burdening healthcare systems. Sedentary lifestyles and poor dietary choices contribute to this epidemic. However, there's hope in the simple yet powerful act of moving our bodies.

The Power of Everyday Physical Activity

Everyday physical activity doesn't necessarily mean grueling gym sessions or intense workouts. It can be as simple as taking a brisk walk, dancing to your favorite tunes, or engaging in activities you genuinely enjoy. This chapter explores various forms of movement, emphasizing the accessibility and inclusivity of physical activity for individuals of all fitness levels.

Breaking Down Barriers

For many, the idea of exercise may be daunting, and overcoming these barriers is a crucial aspect of the battle against obesity. We discuss practical tips to overcome common obstacles such as time constraints, lack of motivation, and perceived physical limitations. By addressing these challenges, individuals can gradually integrate movement into their lives.

Personalizing Your Approach

Finding Your Exercise Bliss involves discovering activities that resonate with your interests and preferences. Whether it's cycling through scenic routes, practicing yoga, or engaging in team sports, there's a myriad of options to explore. Tailoring the approach to individual preferences increases the likelihood of adherence and long-term success in maintaining a physically active lifestyle.

The Psychological Impact

Past the actual advantages, standard activity significantly affects mental prosperity We explore the psychological aspects of embracing physical activity, including stress reduction, improved mood, and increased cognitive function. Understanding these positive effects can serve as powerful motivators in the journey toward a healthier, more active life.

Building Habits That Last

Long-term success in the fight against obesity hinges on establishing sustainable habits. We provide practical advice on building routines that withstand the test of time, ensuring that physical activity becomes an ingrained and enjoyable part of daily life.

Creating a Supportive Environment

Encircling yourself with a strong local area can fundamentally influence your journey Whether it's finding workout buddies, joining fitness classes, or connecting with online communities, a supportive environment fosters accountability and motivation.

Monitoring Progress

Tracking progress is a vital component of any health journey. We discuss effective methods for monitoring physical activity, celebrating milestones, and adapting goals to ensure continued growth.

Ultimately, this chapter advocates for a holistic approach to combating obesity. Embracing everyday physical activity goes hand in hand with nutritional choices, mental well-being, and overall lifestyle adjustments. By addressing these aspects collectively, individuals can foster lasting change and significantly improve their health.

"Move, Groove, and Improve" serves as a roadmap for individuals seeking to fight against obesity by incorporating daily physical activity into their lives. Through personalized approaches, overcoming barriers, and embracing the joy of movement, readers can embark on a transformative journey towards a healthier, more active lifestyle.

Chapter 5: Mindful Eating Mastery

Understanding Mindful Eating:

1. Define mindful eating as the practice of being fully present during meals, paying attention to sensations, emotions, and the act of eating itself.

Savor Every Bite:

2. Encourage readers to engage their senses, savoring the flavors and textures of each bite. Highlight the satisfaction that comes from truly enjoying food.

Listening to Hunger Cues:

3. Emphasize the importance of listening to the body's hunger and fullness cues. Guide readers to distinguish between physical hunger and emotional cravings.

The Power of Eating with Awareness:

Conscious Food Choices:

1. Discuss the impact of making conscious and informed food choices. Provide tips on reading food labels, understanding nutritional values, and opting for whole, nutrient-dense foods.

Slow and Steady Wins the Race:

2. Explore the benefits of eating at a slower pace. Explain how this allows the

body to recognize fullness, preventing overeating, and aiding digestion.

Mealtime Environment:

3. Highlight the significance of creating a positive and relaxed mealtime environment. Discuss the impact of sitting down at a table, minimizing distractions, and enjoying meals in a calm setting.

Navigating Emotional Eating Habits:

Identifying Triggers:

1. Guide readers in recognizing emotional triggers that lead to overeating. Encourage keeping a journal to identify patterns and emotions associated with eating.

Healthy Coping Mechanisms:

2. Introduce alternative, healthier coping mechanisms for dealing with stress, boredom, or emotional challenges. This could include exercise, meditation, or engaging in hobbies.

Building Emotional Resilience:

3. Discuss the role of building emotional resilience in overcoming emotional eating. Encourage readers to seek support and develop strategies for managing stress in a constructive manner.

mastering mindful eating and understanding the power of eating with awareness can be pivotal in the fight against obesity. By incorporating these easy steps into daily life, individuals can foster a healthier relationship with food, make informed choices, and navigate emotional eating habits successfully. Remember, the journey to combat obesity begins with a mindful and intentional approach to eating, paving the way for lasting health and well-being.

Chapter 6: Hydration for Health

Hydration plays a crucial role in the fight against obesity, contributing significantly to weight management. In this comprehensive guide, we'll delve into the importance of water in maintaining a healthy weight and explore enjoyable and straightforward methods to stay adequately hydrated.

Maintaining optimal hydration levels is essential for overall health and well-being. Water is a fundamental component of the human body, comprising a significant percentage of our cells, tissues, and organs. Adequate hydration supports various bodily functions, including digestion, nutrient absorption, temperature regulation, and toxin elimination.

When it comes to combating obesity, water can be a powerful ally. Consuming water before meals can promote a feeling of fullness, reducing the likelihood of overeating. Additionally, staying well-hydrated enhances metabolism, aiding in the efficient burning of calories. Proper hydration also supports physical activity, which is a key component of any weight management strategy.

Water's Role in Weight Management
Understanding the relationship between water and weight management is crucial for anyone seeking to combat obesity. Firstly, water is a calorie-free beverage, making it an excellent alternative to sugary drinks that contribute to excess calorie intake. By replacing high-calorie beverages with water, individuals can create a calorie deficit, an essential aspect of weight loss.

Furthermore, dehydration can sometimes be mistaken for hunger, leading to unnecessary snacking and increased calorie consumption. Regular water intake helps prevent this confusion, ensuring that the body's signals for hunger and thirst are accurately interpreted.

Water also plays a vital role in the breakdown and absorption of nutrients. Proper hydration supports digestive processes, maximizing the body's ability to extract essential nutrients from food. This, in turn, contributes to overall health and can assist in weight management by promoting a balanced diet.

Fun and Easy Ways to Stay Hydrated
Making hydration enjoyable and convenient is key to incorporating it seamlessly into daily life. Here are some fun and easy strategies to stay hydrated:

1. **Flavored Water**: Infuse water with natural flavors by adding slices of fruits,

such as lemon, cucumber, or berries. This adds a refreshing twist without the added sugars found in many flavored beverages.

2. **Hydration Apps:** Utilize smartphone apps that remind you to drink water regularly. These apps often come with customizable settings to suit your personal preferences and lifestyle.

3. **Hydration Stations:** Keep reusable water bottles within easy reach throughout your home, workplace, and car. Having water readily available makes it more likely that you'll sip throughout the day.

4. **Herbal Teas**: Incorporate herbal teas into your routine. While not all teas count towards your daily water intake, they contribute to overall hydration and offer diverse flavors without added calories.

5. **Water-Rich Foods**: Consume foods with high water content, such as watermelon, cucumber, and celery. These not only contribute to hydration but also provide essential nutrients and fiber.

6. **Hydration Challenges**: Turn staying hydrated into a game by setting daily challenges or goals. This could include finishing a certain number of water bottles or trying different infused water combinations.

7. **Sip with Every Snack**: Whenever you have a snack, make it a habit to take a few sips of water. This not only aids in hydration but also helps control portion sizes and promotes mindful eating.

8. **Create a Routine**: Establish a hydration routine by drinking a glass of water at specific times, such as upon waking, before meals, and before bedtime.

Consistency is key to forming healthy habits.

By incorporating these simple and enjoyable strategies, individuals can make hydration a seamless part of their daily lives, contributing to their overall health and supporting their efforts in combating obesity.

recognizing the importance of hydration in weight management is a crucial step in the fight against obesity. By understanding how water impacts the body and implementing fun and easy ways to stay hydrated, individuals can make significant strides towards achieving and maintaining a healthy weight. Remember, small changes in hydration habits can lead to substantial benefits in the long run.

Chapter 7: Social Smartness

In the modern era, where sedentary lifestyles and unhealthy dietary habits prevail, combating obesity has become a pressing concern. This article explores practical and accessible strategies to foster a healthier lifestyle, focusing on the significance of social smartness, making healthy choices in social settings, and effectively managing celebrations and peer pressure.

1.Build a Supportive Network:
Surround yourself with individuals who prioritize health and wellness. A supportive network can positively

influence your choices and provide encouragement on your journey to combat obesity.

1. **Engage in Group Activities**: Participate in group fitness classes, sports, or recreational activities. The social aspect not only makes exercise enjoyable but also creates a sense of accountability, motivating you to stay committed.

2. **Utilize Social Media Positively**: Leverage social media platforms to connect with like-minded individuals, join fitness communities, and share your progress. The online community can offer valuable insights, tips, and encouragement.

Healthy Choices in Social Settings:

1. **Mindful Eating**: Practice mindful eating during social gatherings. Pay attention to portion sizes, savor each bite, and be conscious of hunger and fullness cues. This can prevent overindulgence and promote healthier food choices.

2. **Opt for Nutrient-Rich Options:** When faced with food choices at social events, prioritize nutrient-dense options. Choose lean proteins, whole grains, fruits, and vegetables over processed and high-calorie foods.

3. **Stay Hydrated:** Drinking water before and during social events can help control appetite and prevent overeating. Opting for water over sugary beverages also reduces calorie intake.

Handling Celebrations and Peer Pressure:

1. **Set Realistic Goals**: Establish realistic goals for yourself, especially during celebrations. Understand that occasional indulgence is acceptable, but moderation is key to maintaining a healthy lifestyle.

2. **Communicate Your Goals**: Share your health and fitness goals with friends and family. Communicating your intentions can garner support and reduce external pressures to engage in unhealthy behaviors.

3. **Offer Healthy Alternatives**: If you're hosting an event, provide a variety of healthy food options. This not only supports your personal journey but also encourages your guests to make nutritious choices.

Combatting obesity involves not only individual efforts but also a strategic approach to navigating social situations. By cultivating social smartness, making healthy choices in social settings, and effectively managing celebrations and peer pressure, individuals can pave the way towards a healthier and more sustainable lifestyle. Embracing these easy steps not only benefits personal well-being but also contributes to a collective effort in addressing the global challenge of obesity.

Chapter 8: Support System Strategies

Obesity is a complex health issue affecting millions globally. Tackling it requires a multifaceted approach, and one effective aspect is creating a supportive environment. Support systems play a pivotal role in the journey towards a healthier lifestyle. By implementing strategies that foster accountability and connecting with like-minded individuals, combating obesity becomes more manageable.

Family Involvement:

1. Engaging family members in the journey can provide a strong support system. Shared meal planning, regular physical

activities, and open communication about health goals create a collaborative atmosphere.

Professional Guidance:

2. Seeking guidance from healthcare professionals, such as nutritionists and fitness trainers, ensures a personalized approach. Their expertise helps in formulating realistic plans tailored to individual needs.

Technology Integration:

3. Utilizing health and fitness apps can enhance accountability. Tracking daily activities, food intake, and progress motivates individuals to stay on course and provides tangible data for adjustments.

Building Accountability into Your Routine:

Goal Setting:

1. Clearly defined, achievable goals act as milestones. Breaking down long-term objectives into smaller, manageable steps provides a sense of accomplishment and helps in sustaining motivation.

Regular Check-Ins:

2. Establishing routine check-ins, either with oneself or a support network, fosters accountability. Reflecting on progress and challenges allows for adjustments, preventing setbacks.

Documentation:

3. Keeping a journal detailing daily habits, meals, and physical activities provides a visual record. Reviewing this documentation helps identify patterns and areas for improvement.

Connecting with Like-minded Individuals:

Online Communities:

1. Joining virtual communities focused on healthy living allows for shared experiences and advice. Platforms like social media or specialized forums provide a space for encouragement and motivation.

Group Activities:

2. Participating in group fitness classes or sports not only promotes physical

activity but also cultivates a sense of camaraderie. Sharing the journey with others creates a supportive and uplifting environment.

Support Groups:

3. Local or online support groups specifically addressing obesity offer a space for individuals facing similar challenges to share insights, successes, and setbacks. This sense of community can be a powerful motivator.

an effective strategy for combating obesity involves establishing a robust support system. By incorporating family, seeking professional guidance, leveraging technology, and connecting with like-minded individuals, individuals can build a sustainable framework for healthier living. Creating accountability through goal setting, regular check-ins, and documentation further strengthens the foundation for long-term success. Together, these strategies provide a comprehensive and practical approach to navigate the complexities of obesity and work towards a healthier, more fulfilling life.

Chapter 9: Conclusion

In conclusion, the battle against obesity is a complex yet crucial journey that demands comprehensive lifestyle changes and societal awareness. As we reflect on the easy steps to fight against this pervasive issue, it becomes evident that a holistic approach is necessary. In a world dominated by sedentary lifestyles and processed foods, making informed choices about nutrition and physical activity is paramount.

One of the fundamental strategies in this fight is fostering a deep understanding of nutrition. Embracing a balanced diet rich in fruits, vegetables, lean proteins, and whole grains lays the foundation for a healthier life. Portion control and mindful eating further contribute to weight management, emphasizing the importance of savoring each bite and recognizing the body's signals of hunger and satiety.

Equally crucial is the integration of regular physical activity into daily routines. Whether it's a brisk walk, a workout session, or engaging in recreational sports, consistent exercise not only burns calories but also improves overall well-being. Encouraging communities to embrace active living, with accessible parks and recreational spaces, promotes a culture of fitness and counters the sedentary norms prevalent in modern society.

Beyond personal lifestyle changes, the fight against obesity extends to societal structures and policies. Advocating for healthier school meals, implementing nutrition education programs, and creating urban environments that prioritize walkability all play pivotal roles. Governments, communities, and businesses must collaborate to shape an environment that supports healthier choices, making it easier for individuals to maintain a balanced lifestyle.

Addressing the psychological aspects of obesity is equally essential. Breaking free from the stigma associated with body image and weight issues is crucial for fostering a positive and supportive atmosphere. Encouraging open dialogue about mental health, body positivity, and self-acceptance contributes to a society that values well-being over unrealistic beauty standards.

In this journey, support networks become invaluable. Family, friends, and communities play pivotal roles in creating an environment where individuals feel empowered to make healthier choices. Group activities, such as cooking classes or fitness clubs, can strengthen bonds and provide a collective sense of purpose in the pursuit of a healthier lifestyle.

While the path to overcoming obesity may be challenging, the long-term benefits are profound. Improved physical health, enhanced mental well-being, and a reduced risk of associated health conditions are all achievable outcomes. As individuals commit to making positive changes, they contribute not only to their personal well-being but also to a global shift towards a healthier and more sustainable future.

In conclusion, the fight against obesity is a shared responsibility that requires dedication, education, and a collective commitment to change. By embracing a holistic approach that addresses lifestyle choices, societal structures, and psychological well-being, we can build a healthier and more resilient world, where individuals thrive and obesity becomes a rare exception rather than the norm. Let us embark on this journey together, empowering one another to make lasting, positive choices for a healthier future.